The Way of the Cross
for Those Who Are HIV Positive
and for Those Living with AIDS

Br. Ronald (Ted) Tokarz, O.F.M.

A Liturgical Press Book

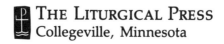

THE LITURGICAL PRESS
Collegeville, Minnesota

Cover design by Fred Petters.

For the inspiration in preparing this work, I would like to thank Sr. Kay Lawlor, M.M.M., pastoral care coordinator, Kitova Hospital, Masaka, Uganda, for her meditation "The Way of the Cross" published in *Catholic International,* volume 2, number 20.

Introduction

Jesus, we come to you in this time of trial and helplessness. You have shown us how we are to bear our daily crosses by your own example. We who are living with AIDS can accept that, but we turn to you and ask for the strength to be able to do so, and comfort when the pain and suffering become overpowering. We identify with you, for you too have shared our experiences of rejection, abandonment, and depression. We have been smitten with a dreadful disease that will eventually overcome our bodies, but which will never destroy our faith and hope in your love for us, unless we allow it to do so. We will walk the Way of the Cross with you and in return, we ask that you walk our Way of the Cross with us.

I
Jesus Is Condemned to Death

Leader: The young man sat down in shock, unable to speak. His hands were trembling and tears began to trickle down his cheeks. He had just been told that he had tested HIV positive. "I'm going to die," he tearfully repeats, "I'm going to die."

Leader: O Compassionate Savior, look graciously upon our affliction,

People: and deliver us by the love you have for us.

All: Lord, help me to bear my fate in the spirit of acceptance and trust. Help me to prepare myself for my own personal Way of the Cross. Look upon me with compassion and be my strength and comfort when the way becomes difficult and the burden, overpowering. I ask this in the name of Jesus who accepted the sentence of death because he loved me so much.

II
Jesus Takes Up His Cross

Leader: People who are HIV positive are weighed down
not only with the knowledge of what this
dreadful disease can do, but they also are beginning to experience the physical, psychological,
and spiritual devastation and havoc it causes in
their bodies and in their beings. How can they
explain this to their loved ones, to their fami-
lies, to their friends? It is so difficult, the burden so great. They realize that this Way of the
Cross will lead to their Calvary.

Leader: O Compassionate Savior, look graciously upon
our affliction,

People: **and deliver us by the love you have for us.**

All: **Lord, I feel so depressed and abandoned.
How can I face those I love and those who
love me? Must I bear this cross alone? Won't
you help them to understand? I need their
understanding, I need their love now more
than ever before. They can help to remove
the sting and the "aloneness" of my suffering. I ask this in the name of Jesus who
accepted his cross out of love for me.**

✝

III
Jesus Falls the First Time

Leader: Many people who are HIV positive, as well as many of those living with AIDS, are forced to walk alone. They feel abandoned in times of weakness and need. They fall into depression and give in to anger and resentment. But a loyal friend shows up and helps them to regain sufficient strength to continue the journey. That friend brings hope to fight off the aura of defeat.

Leader: O Compassionate Savior, look graciously upon our affliction,

People: **and deliver us by the love you have for us.**

All: **Lord, help me to follow your example. Help me not to complain even though the pain is great and I begin to feel sorry for myself. Yes, there are times when I become angry and curse others, even you. At such times strengthen me by your example and help me to resume my journey. The road is very difficult. I need others, above all, I need your help! I ask this in the name of Jesus as he fell the first time under the weight of his cross.**

IV
Jesus Meets His Mother

Leader: Like Jesus, who met his mother on his way to the cross, so too the person who is HIV positive is anxious about meeting his/her mother and the reaction that will follow this meeting. Both realize that the journey towards death has begun. The HIV positive person seeks comfort and understanding. As they meet, a look of love and pain passes between them. The cry "I'm HIV positive!" fills the air. She takes her child into her arms and presses him/her to her heart. And both weep.

Leader: O Compassionate Savior, look graciously upon our affliction,

People: and deliver us by the love you have for us.

All: Lord, just as the presence of your mother was both a source of comfort and pain to you, I beg you to allow her to love and comfort me, for I too, am her child. Also, let others reach out to me in love and compassion. Let them care enough to relieve the pain of my suffering and be there when I need them. I ask this in the name of Jesus and his loving Mother.

V
Simon Helps Jesus Carry His Cross

Leader: People who are HIV positive begin to realize
that they have many decisions to make. How
can they carry on? Their lives are changing.
They slowly will become dependent upon
others. They want to make their fears and anxi-
eties known to their loved ones, to their relatives and friends. They look for an outstretched
hand and a grip that reassures them that
someone does care.

Leader: O Compassionate Savior, look graciously upon
our affliction,
People: **and deliver us by the love you have for us.**

All: **Lord, I have such a fear of all doors being
shut to me. I'm afraid to seek someone to
help me for fear that no one will be there. I
must begin to learn to rely on the goodness
of others. I fear rejection, I fear abuse.
Please inspire my loved ones to be open to
my needs and to the "little things" that
must be done for me. I ask this in the name
of Jesus who allowed Simon to help carry his
cross.**

VI

Veronica Wipes the Face of Jesus

Leader: Many people with AIDS lie in their beds, too weak to take care of or to clean themselves. Their clothing is dirty and soiled. They exist in an atmosphere of utter despair and abandonment. They hope that someone will come to help them, and sometimes a caring person does appear who washes them and changes their soiled clothing. The eyes of the person with AIDS respond with gratitude and a smile.

Leader: O Compassionate Savior, look graciously upon our affliction,
People: and deliver us by the love you have for us.

All: Lord, let me leave my imprint upon the world around me. Let those I have met and continue to meet remember me not because I am among the AIDS statistics, but because I am learning to live bravely with AIDS without bitterness, without anger and without blaming. I ask this in the name of Jesus who allowed Veronica to minister to him.

VII
Jesus Falls a Second Time

Leader: People living with AIDS are capable of contracting many infections, all of which attack the body and weaken it. Diarrhea becomes a problem. Eating habits worsen until food no longer is appealing. Sleep doesn't come easily, breathing becomes harder. As the disease progresses, the person with AIDS becomes weaker, more dependent and more fearful.

Leader: O Compassionate Savior, look graciously upon our affliction,

People: **and deliver us by the love you have for us.**

All: **Lord, I am beginning to feel the weight of this disease. It attacks me from all sides. I can feel myself getting weaker. I know that I am no longer in control. I look to others for the strength to continue and not give up. I refuse to become an object of pity. I am not totally incapacitated, for I still have the will to get up and continue my way of the cross. It is not time yet! I must go on. Help me Lord, help me by your second fall, help me!**

✝

VIII
Jesus Meets the Weeping Women

Leader: Jane is an abused wife; Elena and Henny are discriminated against; Doris has an alcoholic husband; Di sells her body in order to feed her children; Kelly is a druggie; Donna is harassed at work—the plight of women and their vulnerability to abuse and to AIDS. They cry out to an insensitive world, a world that does not hear.

Leader: O Compassionate Savior, look graciously upon our affliction,

People: **and deliver us by the love you have for us.**

All: **Lord, help me to be an instrument of your peace. Let this suffering that I undergo be the source by which I can wash away my sins. Help me to tell my story to others, not to elicit sympathy, but to deter others from succumbing to this dreadful disease. Help me to live with my suffering, yes, even to embrace it without shame, without resentment, without guilt, for these only serve to destroy. I ask this in the name of Jesus who, in the midst of his own suffering, comforted the women who cried over him.**

✝

IX
Jesus Falls a Third Time

Leader: My head feels like it is ready to burst; my body is burning with fever; pain racks every limb and every joint. Nothing brings relief or if it does, it is very temporary. I lie on my bed unable to open my eyes because the pain is so intense. As the disease progresses, I am moved from one room to another, and the pain continues. One more step along the way of the cross—my own personal journey toward my Creator and my God.

Leader: O Compassionate Savior, look graciously upon our affliction,
People: **and deliver us by the love you have for us.**

All: **Lord, the journey is long and painful. Please, keep me from despair. Keep me in your love, in your sight. The time is getting shorter. Let me feel your presence each day remaining to me and let this sense of presence strengthen me until the moment we meet, when suffering and pain will be replaced by joy and everlasting bliss. I ask this in the name of Jesus and his third fall under the weight of the cross.**

X

Jesus Is Stripped of His Garments

Leader: People with AIDS are often rejected by many who were once close to them. Thus begins the process of being stripped of all that was once taken for granted. The right to belong is taken away, as well as human dignity. They become an unwanted commodity. Society labels them vile sinners, deviates who righteously deserve their fate. Hands are extended, not in compassion or assistance, but in accusation and hate.

Leader: O Compassionate Savior, look graciously upon our affliction,

People: **and deliver us by the love you have for us.**

All: **Lord, as you were stripped of all your worldly possessions, so too I have been stripped of everything except my faith in you, and even at times, that wavers. I may end up in a hospital bed, pierced with tubes, abandoned, and left to die. Please, Lord, sustain me with your love and your promise of salvation. Be gentle with me Lord, for I hurt so much! I ask this in the name of Jesus whose nakedness was exposed to the gaze of all.**

XI

Jesus Is Nailed to the Cross

Leader: As the disease becomes more pronounced, breathing becomes more difficult and movement more painful. The person with AIDS is at the mercy of those who care for him/her. He/she feels the loss of something very precious, namely, control and independence. The AIDS related infections have nailed him/her to the cross in the form of a bed, and placed him/her at the mercy of another.

Leader: O Compassionate Savior, look graciously upon our affliction,

People: and deliver us by the love you have for us.

All: Lord, you accepted being nailed to the cross. Silently, you endured the abuse and the pain. Help me, Lord, for there are times when I wish to shout out my pain and curse my fate. I wish to blame others and myself, but your example silences me. My friends help me through the painful times. They listen! They understand! They remind me of how much you love me. I ask this in the name of Jesus who suffered the nails for love of me.

XII

Jesus Dies upon the Cross

Leader: John, Dan, Carol, Tim, Don, Sally, Gina, Tracy, and so many others have already died. Chet, Tom, Bill, Susan, Mona, Russ, Larry, and many others are in various stages of AIDS. They too are slowly dying: the body of Jesus is being ravaged by AIDS!

Leader: O Compassionate Savior, look graciously upon our affliction,

People: and deliver us by the love you have for us.

All: Lord, you died upon the cross forgiving those who crucified you. You even promised salvation to the good thief. As my time to depart from this world draws near and you call me to join you in your Kingdom, let me come to you with the love of those who surround me, and who are so much a part of me. I ascend to you on the wings of an eagle, with a body, though broken by this dreadful disease, that will be made whole and beautiful again. I ask this in the name of Jesus who died to save all people.

XIII
Jesus Is Taken Down from the Cross

Leader: The crying begins. The body has finally been overcome by this ravaging disease. It is placed in a shroud and taken to an undertaker who is willing to prepare the body for burial. The companion and the mother of the one who has died of AIDS reach out to touch and caress a friend who will always be remembered, a child whose presence will no longer be there. They look upon the body, someone they love, for the last time.

Leader: O Compassionate Savior, look graciously upon our affliction,

People: and deliver us by the love you have for us.

All: Lord Jesus, your lifeless, torn and bruised body was taken down from the cross and laid in the bosom of your Mother. My body too, emaciated and disfigured by AIDS, will be brought to your Kingdom, where pain and suffering, shame and guilt have been overcome on the tree of the cross. This body will no longer be emaciated, covered with cancerous growths, and its respiratory system will be free of every and all infections. Reach out to me, grasp my hand. Your touch will make me sound and whole. I ask this in the name of Jesus who, in life and in death, found rest in the bosom of his loving Mother.

✝

XIV

Jesus Is Placed in a Tomb

Leader: A grave has been dug. A few relatives and friends (those who are left) come to say their farewells. Many standing around the grave carry this dreadful disease in their bodies. They realize that soon their time will come, but until then, they must continue to walk their individual and personal way of the cross. They must live with AIDS but in the end, they will be the victors. Their intense suffering and excruciating pains are the instruments of their peace.

Leader: O Compassionate Savior, look graciously upon our affliction,

People: **and deliver us by the love you have for us.**

All: **Lord, your suffering has come to an end. You have accomplished your mission of salvation. In three days you will overthrow death and rise again. Death has lost its sting and no longer is the victor. My mission too will come to an end, regardless of my age. I too must accomplish all that was given me to do. Time goes by swiftly! There is still much to be done. Help me Lord, please help me! I ask this in the name of Jesus who had nowhere to lay his head and was buried in a stranger's tomb.**

✝

XV
Resurrection

Leader: The grave only seems to be the end. What
death has actually done is to open the door to
eternal life, a life that knows no tears or experiences any sorrow. In this life, the body was
wasted away by a disease we call AIDS; in eter-
nity, the body will be healthy and beautiful. It
finally took death to overcome this disease.
Death is no longer the victor, but our liberator.
In Jesus, love conquered death and this enabled
everyone, including all of us living with AIDS,
to enjoy and to possess the one for whom and
by whom we were created: God.

.

EMBRACING THE MYSTERY

Prayerful Responses to AIDS

Sebastian Sandys

AIDS and HIV have claimed the lives of many hundreds of thousands of people in our country and elsewhere. As so often happens in times of trouble, people are turning to God—in anger, in confusion, in need, and in help-lessness.

Many of the original contri-butions to this book of reflec-tions are written by people living those feelings, dwelling in the midst of all the pain that AIDS brings. Yet they have been brought closer to God and supported by the love they have found there. This collection is offered in support of those still struggling to find God's presence.

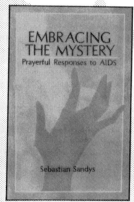

2222-4   Paper, 120 pp., 5 3/8 x 8 1/4, $8.95

Rights: U.S., Canada, Mexico, Central America (except Belize), and Puerto Rico

Phone: **1-800-858-5450** Fax: **1-800-445-5899**

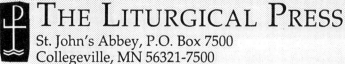

THE LITURGICAL PRESS

St. John's Abbey, P.O. Box 7500
Collegeville, MN 56321-7500